Every Road Has A Bend

The True Story About A Child's Bravery

R. Ashley

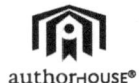

authorHOUSE®

AuthorHouse™ UK Ltd.
500 Avebury Boulevard
Central Milton Keynes, MK9 2BE
www.authorhouse.co.uk
Phone: 08001974150

First published by AuthorHouse 7/18/2007

ISBN: 978-1-4343-2029-2 (sc)

Printed in the United States of America
Bloomington, Indiana

This book is printed on acid-free paper.

Chapter One

Something's Not Right

Our story begins in the year 1996. It is a special day for us; today my wife has just given birth to a beautiful baby boy. He weighs a healthy nine pounds and one ounce, and has blonde hair and blue eyes. He looks so perfect lying in his crib, and soon we take him home to meet his brother's and sister's. Everything is fine, until one day, six months after he was born, things started to change.

It was a hot day and while our son was sitting on my wife's knee, she took his shirt off. I was playing with him and making him laugh, but then my eyes suddenly glanced at his back and my laughter soon stopped! My wife asked, "What's the matter love?" I looked at her and replied, "Our son's back doesn't look right." I begin to feel his back. "It feels strange, there's a bump, and it seems his ribs are out of shape," I said. My wife looked at me in horror. "What could this be? Is our son alright?" she said, "I think we should take him to the doctors straight away" I replied.

When we arrived at the doctors, she removed our son's shirt. We could see by the expression on her face that there was something seriously wrong. She says, "I am not sure what it is, but I will have to send you to the hospital." Our hearts sink, and we begin to get very worried. "What could this be? What is happening to our son?" we wondered. A few weeks pass by, and then we get an appointment to see a doctor at the hospital. Our son has numerous x-rays, and we are taken into a small room. We are told, "Your son has a curved spine, and it's a condition called scoliosis" …we begin to cry, and ask "what will happen to our son?" the doctor says, "he will have to go to a hospital in Nottingham which specialise in his condition," we ask him, "Will he need surgery?" The doctor replies, "That is a possibility."

A few weeks later our son goes to see a spinal surgeon at a Nottingham hospital, he says "I have checked all of your son's x-rays, and he doe's have a curvature of the spine." We get very upset and begin to cry. "He is only six months old?" we say, "how can this happen?" The surgeon tries to comfort us and replies "because he is young, I might be able to control the curve by putting him into a plastic body brace, which he must wear for twenty four hours per day." We look at each other and agree to give it a try, we take his advice hoping that it will control the curve and it doesn't get any worse.

It has been two years now and the jacket has done no good. The curve has steadily got worse, and the surgeon says, "I am sorry, your son's curve is progressing fast and he will have to have surgery. We will have to operate on his side and remove a rib, and then we turn him over and operate on his back to loosen his spine." We feel numb inside and we cannot even think straight. "He will also need rods, screws and wires attached to his spine to help straighten it," says the surgeon. My wife starts to cry, so I put my arms around her, she is sobbing on my shoulder, and I begin to cry also. We cannot believe that our baby has to have major surgery; we slowly calm down and take the lonely drive back home, not knowing what the future may hold.

When we arrived home we are feeling sick in our stomachs; we keep thinking "why?" he's only a child, the youngest of our five children. "Why doe's he have to go through this at such a young age?" Our son is asleep now in his bed; we hold each other... crying, until our eyes slowly close.

We have been told it can take up to two years before the surgery can take place. Our son needs to be a little older and there has to be an intensive care bed available, so it looks like a few more years in the plastic jacket.

It is now the 4th April 2001. Our son is now four years old, and we are travelling to the hospital today which is twenty miles away from our home. When we arrived, the nurse showed us to his bed. Our son is happily playing with some toys, but tomorrow he will be having the first stage of his operations, he will have the second stage in two weeks time. Our son plays for most of the night, then soon settles down and slowly falls asleep. My wife will be sleeping next to him, and I will sleep upstairs in the parent's room. I kiss my wife and son goodnight and make my way upstairs, worrying about what tomorrow may hold. As I lay on my bed in this lonely room, I start thinking about tomorrow's operation. All different thoughts are shooting through my mind, I begin to cry…I am sobbing, and I cannot control myself. My body is shaking, and my head is throbbing. I keep asking myself "why?" he's only four years old, "why?" does he have to go through this. I am tossing and turning all night and didn't get much sleep. The night soon passed and I woke up and looked at my watch. It is now 6.30am and time to go to my wife and son.

When I arrived at our son's bedside, I looked towards my wife. I can see the worry on her face and the tears in her eyes; we hold each others hands, trying to comfort each other. We look across at our son, and he's looking straight at us. We can feel the tears building up inside our eyes, so we stand up and look out of the window; we don't want to get our son upset. All of a sudden we can hear voices behind us; the nurses are here to take our son to surgery. He is looking at us, so we take deep breaths fighting back the tears, but it's very hard, seeing him sitting on the bed in his little white gown. We try to talk to him, and reassure him that everything will be fine, but he is not listening and begins to cry. The nurses are trying to calm him down, and soon we begin to walk down the lonely corridors. Holding our son's hands, and with tears dripping down our cheeks we arrive at the operation theatre. The doctors try to put our son to sleep, but he is struggling and getting very upset, we both calm him down and his eyes slowly begin to close. We both kiss our son, and leave him in the surgeon's hands, saying as we leave… "Take care of him." We hold each other tightly as we slowly walk back to the ward. We are crying all the way, and we hope that everything goes well.

When we get back to the ward, we sit in the lonely parent's room. My wife is crying, and I am sitting there, staring at the floor, "why our son?" we ask each other "he's so young to have to go through major surgery," we cannot stop the tears, and we sit in that room for ages. I look at my watch and say to my wife "it's been over five hours now, why is it taking so long? Something's not right?" we both begin to panic. Suddenly the door swings open and a nurse enters, she says "everything is fine, it's all over, you can go to intensive care to see your son." We smile a little and quickly go upstairs to his bedside.

When we arrived at his bedside, it was such a shock to see him lying there with wires and tubes everywhere. His face is swollen and he has a halo attached to his head, which is pinned into his skull. They have also loosened his spine ready for the next operation. There are monitors everywhere, and every time one bleeps we look at the nurse, but she reassures us that everything is fine. We were told about the risks involved and are looking at his arms and legs; we are praying that he moves them. I can see my wife looking for any movement at all, she asks the nurse "has he moved his legs?" the nurse carefully touches him, and to our relief he moves all of his limbs. Soon afterwards he wakes up and talks to us, we are so happy that everything went well and we stay with our son all night. When he went back to sleep and was comfortable, we quietly went to get some sleep ourselves… We are so glad that today is over.

The next day we went to see our son. He is still fast asleep, so we hold his hand. All of a sudden! The monitor starts to bleep… it won't stop! We are looking at the nurse and she seems very concerned. She is looking around for help, and it looks like his heart rate is dropping. My legs are feeling weak and my hearts pounding. My wife is squeezing my hand and I can see the worry on her face… we are terrified! "What's happening?" we asked. The nurse doesn't say anything, but she looks very worried. Just then to everyone's relief the bleeping stopped, and his heart rate is returning back to normal. It was such a shock for all of us.

The next day we are sitting next to our son, who is still asleep. All of a sudden he wakes up and is pulling at the tube in his mouth, he pulls it straight out and gasps for air. He is now breathing by himself. Throughout the day he improves, and is soon sent downstairs to the high dependency ward. My wife says to the nurse "don't you think it is too soon to take him out of intensive care, he's just had major spine surgery?" The nurse replies "it's alright, it is best for him, and will help him recover faster." But as soon as we arrived in the ward, our son starts shouting loudly "HELP ME UP! HELP ME UP!" his eyes are staring and he is grabbing the bed covers… we cannot stop him! My wife is crying and the nurses are rushing to help. This carries on for nearly an hour. Then… all of a sudden…he stops, and he's back to normal. We asked him "what happened?" but he knew nothing about it, he couldn't remember anything. The nurse takes us to one side and says, "It must be the combination of drugs we have to give him" we are glad that our son is alright, but we were very worried.

I have just been refused permission to sleep, because they need the parent's room. I don't want to leave our son because he has just had major surgery; I have to be near him. So I decided to sleep in my car. It was a cold night, I was freezing and shaking, I am sitting there, staring at the wall in front of me. I keep thinking about my wife and son and I need to be with them… I begin to cry. It is no good I can't get any sleep, so I get out of my car and go to the hospital restaurant and order a cup of coffee. It is now 2am, and I am sitting all alone in this empty restaurant just staring into my cup, my head is throbbing and the tears are beginning to flow yet again. All of a sudden I look up to see a lady standing in front of me, she says, "I am sorry sir but I have to close now," so I slowly get up and walk out. I don't know where to go or what to do; I walk around the empty hospital corridors. I am in a daze and I can't think straight. I walk for hours and hours and when I look at my watch it is 4am, I have to see my wife and son, I need to be near them both. I make my way back to the ward and knock quietly on the door; the nurse opens the door and lets me enter. I go and sit next to my wife and son, who are fast asleep, and I sit quietly in the chair trying not to disturb them. I feel a lot better now that I am near both of them.

Later that day the nurse comes to take the tube out of our son's side, which goes into his lungs to help drain the fluids; our son is crying and getting very upset. We try to calm him down and the nurse pulls quickly on the tube, he lets out a loud scream and it's all over. He is such a brave boy and copes well.

The next day he is moved into the children's ward. The halo attached to his head looks barbaric but is important to help get his spine straight. The nurses come and put weights onto the rope which is attached to his halo. He will have 1lb attached every day for the next ten days, and then he will have the second stage of his operations. The first operation was to loosen his spine and take some bone away. I am not allowed to sleep again, but I am tired and need some rest, so I decided to drive home. It is pouring down, the rain is lashing against my window and I have tears in my eyes. I cannot see the road properly, but I make it home safely.

When I arrived home, I opened my front door to see our neighbour standing in front of me. She asked me about our son, and I tell her "he's doing fine." She is helping us by looking after our home in such a difficult time. I managed to get some sleep, but soon I was woken by the birds chirping outside. I got into my car and drove back to the hospital, hoping that everything was alright throughout the night. When I arrived I checked on our son who seems fine, but my wife looks tired and could do with a rest, but she will not leave his side.

Later in the day my mother and sister arrive. My mother is getting very emotional and upset, she begins to cry. I try to comfort her, but then my sister starts crying also. I hold them both and explain that our son is alright, "please don't cry in front of him, he will get upset," I said. They calm down and give him some presents. Our son is happy and they stay all day. The nurse tells me I am not allowed to stay again so it looks like another night in my car, I managed to get some sleep but it was not very comfortable.

The next day I walked back to the ward; my wife and son had a good night, and soon the nurse comes to remove the tube from his bladder. She also brings a wheelchair with a pulley system attached; it looks weird, but is to help him sit up straight. Our son has been in bed for a week now, and he will be glad to get out. We try him in his chair but he begins to cry, it is very difficult for him because he has all these weights pulling him up by his head. Awhile later he is in the chair and does well for his first time. The nurse talks to us and is worried that he hasn't been to the toilet for eight hours, and they want to put the tube back in. We asked her to wait a while and soon afterwards he was able to go. That night I drove home, I was exhausted and needed some sleep. My wife will sleep next to our son again, she will not leave him.

The next day we asked to see a social worker to help me get a room, we have to be near our son, and there is also a staff shortage. She said she will look into it. We cannot understand why the nurses do not come to this part of the ward often; it gets very boring in here, and where are the nurses? It's been two hours and not one nurse has checked on our son which we think is terrible. A few days later a nurse comes to give our son a wash in his bed, but while wiping his face, the towel gets tangled around the halo our son is wearing, and the nurse pulls on the towel. Our son shouts out in pain, "STOP!" we shouted, "We will wash him ourselves!" There was not enough care and attention taken by this nurse. Later he came to apologise, he told us, "he was sorry, he only comes in to help out, and he is a hairdresser by trade." We don't know if it was due to the staff shortage. Some of the other children are getting infections and have to go back for surgery to be washed out; we are starting to get very worried.

A few days later the sister came to talk to me, she couldn't believe that I had been sleeping in my car and offered me a place to stay. Apparently there was a residence block where I could have stayed which nobody had bothered to tell me about. Our son had an uncomfortable night and was in a lot of pain, later in the day he won an Easter egg in the raffle and that cheered him up a little. Our family and friends also visit today and our son is showing off and making everybody laugh. The nurses are still adding one pound in weight to the pulley system attached to his halo. Our son enjoys himself today and soon it is night time and he's fast asleep.

The following day when I arrived I was told that our son had been sick in the night but was fine afterwards, so they removed the tube from his neck; he will feel more comfortable now, it's just a shame about the nurses. It's been three hours now and we have only seen one nurse, who came to take our son's temperature. We know they have a difficult job, but they still should check on our son. My wife looks tired, she hasn't left our son's side at all; she has never been home or left him. I love her very much and ask her to have a break but she will not leave his bedside.

The next day when I arrive our son is already awake. My wife seems happier and our son is watching television. It makes us smile in the morning when everyone arrives; they all seem to swoop in at the same time. Changing the beds, making the breakfast, washing patients, doctors doing their daily checks. Then they all just disappear, just as quickly as they arrived. We have just spoken to the surgeon and he says "everything went well." It's the first time we have seen him in twelve days and only because we bumped into him in the corridor. Our son is in his wheelchair today and has nine pounds of weight attached to his halo, which is pulling his spine straighter. We decided to go to the hospital restaurant, but as soon as we opened the door, people started staring. Our son is getting very upset…do they realise what they are doing?

We have just spoken to the surgeon; he says he is pleased because he has reduced the curve from 74 degrees to 40 degrees and hopes to reduce it even further on the next operation. The last weight has now been placed on our sons halo traction, and tomorrow he will be having the second stage of his operations… Then we will have to go through it all again.

Our son is asleep in his bed. My wife and I are looking out of the window; we can see all the cars driving by. People doing their everyday things, some with no cares in the world, but our lives have been on hold for the last two weeks and will be for a couple more. The sun is shining outside but not for us, we are still unhappy and sad and want it all to be over with, so we can try to get back to a normal life again. We look at our son sleeping in his bed, looking very comfortable and peaceful. But tomorrow will be another big day.

It is very hard for us, especially when they told us about the risks involved. When they sat us down and explained what would happen, and what could happen if things go wrong. It was very hard, and very emotional. But we couldn't leave our son like that, his spine would have just got worse, and his health would have suffered in the future. So we decided we would have to try and stop the curvature from progressing. We have to think about his future.

Chapter Two

Our Tears Begin Again

It is now 6am on Thursday morning. The nurses are already here, putting the little white gown on our son, but this time he's getting very upset because he knows what's going to happen, and he's shouting at them "TAKE IT OFF!" Another nurse is putting wires onto his head and cream onto his hands, our son keeps shouting "I DON'T WANT A NEEDLE!" We try to comfort our son, but my wife is crying and getting upset also, so I hold her as we walk beside our son down to the theatre. It is very hard for us because our son is really upset and crying all the way down to the operation theatre, we walk beside his bed on that same lonely route. We kiss our son again as his eyes slowly close. The next operation begins…and so do our tears.

It has been six hours now and we haven't heard anything; we are starting to panic again. We asked a nurse to ring the theatre, she returns a few moments later and said "he is still down there." My wife looks shattered and tired, her eyes are red with all the crying and my head is throbbing, we hope everything is alright; it has been such along time. One hour later we get told to go to intensive care, our son is lying in his bed again, all wired up and his face is swollen. He stays asleep all night and seems comfortable, we sit holding his hands until late at night, then we go to try and get some sleep ourselves.

The next day he was complaining of pain in the night and was very uncomfortable, which is understandable for what he has been through. He has had wires, screws and rods attached to his spine. We still cannot believe how fast he is moved to the high dependency ward again, and just two hours later he is moved again to the children's ward, but at least he's happier now and can watch television. I have just spoken to a man whose son has fallen through a roof, he is in intensive care and I hope he's alright. His mother has told me that the doctors have found out he has a heart defect and must operate straight away. She says "it could have been a blessing in disguise, because nobody knew he had anything wrong with his heart." I hope everything goes well for them; they seem such a nice family. Our son has a lot of back pain through the evening and the nurse gives him some medicine. Afterwards he soon settles down and goes to sleep; I kiss my wife and son goodnight and make my way upstairs to my room.

During the night I have such a bad dream, I am sweating and breathing really fast. I shout out in my sleep and wake up shaking. I look at my watch and its 4am, I want to go downstairs to check on our son, but I say to myself "don't be stupid, it's only a dream" so I slowly go back to sleep.

The following day my wife said that our son had a bad night and was in a lot of pain, she was up all night taking care of him. We still think it's too fast how they send them back to the wards so quickly, we asked one of the nurses and she agrees with us. Later that day the nurse removes the large tube which is draining fluid from his lungs, as soon as the nurse touches the tube our son starts to scream. The nurse pulls the tube out and our son lets out a loud scream. It was very upsetting for him but it was over quickly and he soon calms down.

Tomorrow they will try and get him out of bed and into the wheelchair. Our family ring everyday and are such a good help in this difficult time. Even my sister managed to come to the hospital, which was very difficult for her because she has had two terrible tragedies in the past and is still on medication. We understand it must have been very hard for her, and we love her all the same.

A few days later, our son has more tubes and drains removed; he is feeling happier and has been out in his wheelchair. We move the wheelchair further away from him each time to encourage him to walk that little bit more. The nurse says "when he is walking more; he will be able to go home." The physiotherapist comes to help him with his breathing and walking, but he quickly gets tired so we put him to bed and let him rest. The next day the last of the tubes are removed which was in his neck, he begins to cry and is getting upset but he copes well. We cannot believe that the anaesthetist has just come in to check on our son. It was a surprise because it was his day off, what a nice person to come in and check how our son is doing. It was very nice of him and shows how much he cares. Our sister-in-law rings the ward asking if everything is alright, she is very helpful as she is looking after our other four children.

Today our son seems fine, he has been out in his chair, and he has walked quite a bit, everyone thinks he's doing really well. Our family arrive and bring him more presents, he's being spoilt but he doesn't mind. He won't be able to get back into his bed with all those toys over it. The surgeon arrives and is pleased with his progress, we are shown the x-rays and we can see the metal rods, wires and screws attached to his spine, everything looks fine and we hope we don't have to go through this again. Our son has a temperature and the doctors are watching him very closely, and every time he needs turning in bed we have to log roll him, making sure he stays straight at all times. The nurses are making him laugh and looking after him really well. A few nurses come into the ward just to make him smile, which we don't mind because we love it when he's smiling and happy. It can get very depressing sitting in bed all day. Later that day he walks around the ward and the nurses are pleased with his progress. A few hours later he is tired and goes back to bed and soon falls asleep.

We cannot believe that soon we will be going home after three weeks in hospital, that first week was terrible, we never thought any person could cry so much as we did, but I suppose a lot of people go through the same things. We look out of the window, it is dark and cold outside, thundering and lightening, we can hear our son behind us complaining of pain and he wants to be rolled over, so we roll him and he is much happier and falls back to sleep. It has been very stressful for us all over the last three weeks, and to see your own child going through so much is heartbreaking. We are really happy that it is all over, and hope it will be a nice day tomorrow for us and we can all go home.

Today we are going home; the doctors are pleased with his progress. Our son is smiling, he cannot believe that he can finally go home; we begin to get him dressed and take him downstairs in his wheelchair. We say "goodbye" to all the nurses and staff and thank them for looking after our son. It has been a long hard road for us all over the last three weeks, but we are glad that it's all over with, and we are finally going home. We drive home, happy and smiling. I look at our son and he is much happier, then I glance across at my wife and I can see she is happy and relieved that it's all over. The tears have finally stopped. The sun is shinning and we have a pleasant drive home, we even managed to get home before our other four children had come out of school. They opened the front door and were so pleased to see their little brother standing in front of them, they all ran over to hug and kiss him. What a happy sight for us to see, we are now all together again, how it should be. Now at last we can get our lives back on track after such an emotional time.

Chapter Three

This Cannot Be Happening

"OH NO!" We cannot believe what's happened. After all our son has been through, first having one operation to go in through his side, to release bone, remove ribs, and then another operation to remove parts of his spine and to attach wires, screws and rods, after all that. It has now all came away from his spine...after just six months. He has a lot of swelling and redness, and has a puncture wound where the rods have came away from his spine, our son's head has fallen forward and there is a hole in his skin where the rod has penetrated through. We can see the rod through the hole in his skin; we can actually see the rod. And also, it is now a direct route for infection. We cannot believe that after two seven hour operations, it only lasted six months. We thought it was all over with, and we were getting back to normality, but now it looks like we will have to go through it all again.

We had an appointment to see the surgeon, and he said to us "your son will need a small operation to cut the rod down, and stitch the hole back up. In the meantime you have to keep it covered." But we also had to wait nearly four months for the rod to be cut down which was terrible. We couldn't believe why the first operation took over five hours, and only lasted six months. We complained to the hospital and also the media took an interest.

The local newspapers decided to print a story. But we couldn't understand why, after all the operations and all the hours in the operation theatre that the metal rods came away from our son's spine after just six months. We needed some answers.

After complaining to the hospital and the newspapers doing a story, we decided to ask for a more experienced surgeon, one of the top surgeons in scoliosis surgery. We will never forget what he did, he looked at our son and looked towards the floor shaking his head saying "I will have to take everything out and start again from scratch; we cannot leave him like this." We couldn't believe what we have just heard, we are shocked! This means that our son will have to go through it all again, going in through his side, removing ribs, having a halo attached to his head, and being stretched in traction. This cannot be happening to us, and our poor son has to go through it all again, he was really brave to go through what he did the first time around, but to get told it has failed and will have to be re-done is a nightmare to us all.

We don't know what to say to our son, he was so happy when it was all over with when he had the last operations. Now he has to have them all again, we don't know what's going through his mind at this moment in time, he must be terrified!

We haven't had much luck over the years, my wife lost her parents to cancer and I lost my step dad to cancer. We know it happens, and sadly people do lose their parents, but we lost all three parents within five months. We also have an older child who was premature and born three months early. Because of an ambulance strike, my wife and I had to deliver him ourselves on the settee. We had no help whatsoever and had do get through it all ourselves. Luckily there were no complications, but it was still a shock for us, to wake up during the night to find the baby is on the way. Weighing just 3lbs, and spending months in an incubator at the hospital, he has cerebral palsy. But he is seventeen years old now and doing well. But sadly we also had a terrible tragedy in the family… four of my nephews were in an explosion in a garage, one sadly died in the fire and three were badly burned. All the family were at the hospital, trying to comfort our sister, but the tragedy was too bad, and was about to get worse. Just one week later, another one of my sister's son's…my nephew, who was sitting on my knee just a few weeks before, sadly passed away. The pain was unbearable for my sister, and it was a terrible thing to happen. To lose one son in such a bad way was terrible, but to lose another son just a week later, I can't even put it into words. We even had to go out the back door at the hospital because the reporters wouldn't leave us alone. That's when I saw my sister look at our mother, (who she hadn't spoken to for some years) just open her arms and say just one word… "MUM". Our mother rushed over to her and held her tight, and they stood there hugging for ages. We will never ever forget that terrible day.

We are now thinking why do things go bad in life? What have we done? Things always seem to go wrong for us. We went through a lot of pressure and tears, when our own child had that risky operation in the first place, and then the relief we felt when it was all over with. But then to be told he's got to go through it all again, it's hard to cope with and we feel so drained. After my wife and I have a long discussion we decided to let the surgeons try again, and we hope it will last for more than six months this time. We have explained to our son and he seems fine, but he's worried which is understandable.

It's been nearly two years now since our son had his first operation, and we are back at the hospital in the same familiar surroundings. The nurses remember us from last time and are all saying "hello," our son sits on his bed and gets back into the same routine. We notice a boy in here from the last time we were here, he fell over and his rod snapped, which can happen. Our son soon settles down and falls asleep. I help my wife make a bed up next to our son, and I will be sleeping upstairs in that same lonely room, with my emotions and thoughts all over the place. My wife looks sad again, worried sick about the operations to follow.

Today is the day of the operation, the first of two. Our son is getting very upset because he knows what's going to happen. We walk beside him down to the theatre, but this time he is kicking and screaming. We are crying and we have to hold his legs down because he is struggling too much, the doctor is finding it difficult to give him the injection to put him to sleep. They decide to blow some gas into his face to calm him down. It is very hard for us; with the tears dripping down our faces we kiss our son's face as he slowly falls asleep. The surgeon says, "We will look after him." My wife feels faint and needs some fresh air, so we decided to go for a walk. My wife is holding me tight, she is crying while walking down the streets, I stop and hold her saying "everything will be alright, they will take care of him."

Our son has now been in surgery for seven hours and we are getting very concerned, but shortly afterwards he is out and sent to intensive care. Just like the last time we sit holding his hands and watching the monitors, jumping every time we hear a bleep. He has a halo attached to his head, so they can add weights to it and try and stretch his spine. He also has a wound on the other side of his body where they entered from the other side and a huge wound down his back where they tried to correct the curvature.

My wife is happier now she's with him and that the operation is all over with. The nurses say he's doing fine, and we look at our son who seems comfortable and is fast asleep. We hope this time the operations work.

We cannot believe it! We have just been told that our son will have to stay in traction with thirteen pounds of weight pulling on his halo, which is screwed into his skull. Last time it was for ten days, this time they want him in traction for... SIX WEEKS! I don't know how we all cope, especially our son, he's been through so much, and we always look at him and think, God your a brave boy. But like all parents say; we wish it was us and not him, having to go through this. To go through it once was bad enough, but he has to go through it twice. Children show the true courage.

The six weeks are now over with, and it's been very hard for my wife and me to watch our son go through so much. Watching the pain he's been through and the nurses doing their very best to try and cheer him up. Our son seems fine and never seems to complain, children are amazing and some go through terrible things yet they never moan or complain, they are amazing and put us adults to shame. The nurses are great and make him smile, and he has the thirteen pounds of weight attached to his halo, which doesn't seem to bother him much. But he knows that soon he will have to have the second stage of his operations and does seem to be a little upset, though he tries to hide it. We reassure him and try to cheer him up; we like to make him smile. The surgeon arrives and tells us "this time I will attach more rods, screws and wires but also to be certain that his head doesn't fall forward I will attach a clamp to the top of the rods."

Today is the next stage of the operations, our son is getting used to it now and knows what to expect. He does get upset in the operation theatre but soon calms down and we both kiss him again. He is now in their hands for the next seven hours; we still worry and cry until he safely comes back to us… as all parents do. We go through the same routine again and hope that this will be the last operation.

Our son is now out of surgery, and the operation went well. It is very worrying for us and we hope that it's the last operation. We also worry about the scaring on his back, because the doctor said "it gets more difficult when he goes through the same procedure time after time."… We just want it all to end.

It has been a week now and our son looks taller, he seems happier, but something is worrying my wife and me. We can see a bump in-between his shoulders, it may be the clamp to stop him from falling over the top of the rods, so we asked the surgeon and he confirms it is the clamp, he says "hopefully that will stop his head and neck from falling forward."

So once again our son had to go through another set of operations, because the first lot failed. But hopefully now he has the clamp on the end of the rods, this will stop any future problems.

We are now on our way home and happy that it's all over with. Our son is happier too, and just wants to go home and get back to normal. When we arrived home everyone is pleased to see him. The neighbours come out, and all his friends are glad to see him also. They are asking him about his operations, but he's tired and just wants to rest. Our son is much happier now that he's back home, he has been through so much and we hope that he doesn't go through that again. We really do hope that this is the last of the operations.

Chapter Four

Not Again … Please

"OH No! Not again!" Our son has had infections since leaving hospital seven weeks ago. But now, having had one of the top surgeons around, he has again fallen over the top of the rods. His head has fallen forward and you can see the bump on his back is more prominent, he is in no pain but at this moment in time it is hard for us to cope.

My wife and I cry every night and our pillows are soaking wet with the tears, the crying has begun again. We cannot believe that our son has already had one set of unsuccessful operations, they took everything out and started again from the beginning, and now we are being told that this one has failed also. The pressure on us is immense, and we still have to explain to our son that he might have to go through it all yet again.

We are now at the hospital, and the surgeon is looking at our son, he turns to us and we know what he is about to say, we can see it in his face. My wife and I look at each other, not wanting to hear those words yet again... Then the surgeon speaks, saying "I am sorry, we cannot leave him like this, we will have to try again, and it means he will have to go through the same process all over again." My wife looks at me, and I can see that she's holding back her tears, I feel empty inside and our son is looking at us with his big blue eyes. We don't know what to say, we cannot wonder what he is thinking inside. We are not sure if we can take anymore, and as for our son, we don't know if we should put him through it all again.

It is now April 2004, and we have just come home from the hospital, we feel empty and sad. Our son is playing happily at home with his toys, but we have spoken to the surgeon and he wants our son back into hospital by July, so he can once again remove all the metalwork, put him back in traction, stretch his spine, but this time he wants to go further up into the neck area, and maybe use some kind of strut at the front of the spine to help support it.

We cannot believe he has to go through it all again, when is this all going to end! Year after year our son is having major spinal surgery and the stress and strain for us his parents are huge. The operations are very risky to perform, yet our son is having them nearly every year, how much can we all take. If you are a parent you will know what we mean about all the worry and stress, we know it's part of life and comes with being a parent, but when you see your own child laying on that operation table in their little white gowns, their eyes looking at you, and you looking back, trying to hold back your tears so they don't get upset, its very, very hard and very upsetting. Once again we are on the same road as last time, the same routine, and the same tears are about to flow yet again.

We come to a decision to let our son have a rest from all these operations, and we leave it for a year. We have an appointment to see the surgeon in September, and we will listen to what he suggests is best for our son.

It is now September and just over a month ago I had some bad news, my father died suddenly from a heart attack, and we have just received some more bad news. The surgeon wants to operate again next year, but this time he wants to open up our son's chest and go in through the front, as well as the back. He wants to put a strut of bone on the front of his spine to stop him from falling forward. We don't think we can put him through that. It would be like having open heart surgery, going by the heart to the spine, and having it stapled shut afterwards.

We have been crying ever since he told us, even our son was saying in the car on the way home "mum what if they damage my heart," We told him they wouldn't, but a eight year old child shouldn't have to be going through this, never lone thinking about it.

Christmas has come and gone. We love seeing all the children opening their presents, we always make sure they have a good time, and it's nice seeing all their smiling faces. We have a few months before we see the surgeons again, lets hope this time things turn out for the best.

It is now April 2005, and we have just seen the surgeon, just like we expected, our son has to go back into hospital so they can try again to correct his progressing curvature of the spine. The surgeon has just said to us that "in all his twenty years of performing corrective surgery, our son is one of the most unusual cases he has came across," he cannot understand why everything always seems to fail. Let's hope this time it will be a success.

We get very upset with the surgeons and criticize them, but it must be very hard and frustrating for them to do all this risky surgery, only to find that it fails months later.

Our son will have to have more surgery in July, and he knows what to expect now because he's been through it so many times before, and he's also getting older now. We often see him looking in the mirror, thinking about his physical appearance, and he is always checking his posture. He also has swimming lessons at school, but refuses to go because he gets upset when people stare at him.

We have had no news from the hospital for quite awhile, so we decide to treat the children to a family holiday, we haven't been away for nearly eight years, and so the break will do us all good. The children are happy and our son is smiling.

Five days after we booked our holiday, we had to cancel it, because we have just had a phone call from the hospital; they want our son to be admitted in September for more surgery, and then another operation in October. We cannot believe it, the only time we plan to go on holiday and we have to cancel it, but even though our children are upset, our son's health has to come first and the holiday can wait. We have one month now to prepare ourselves for what is going to be more stress, worry, tears and heartache as our son goes for more surgery. We love him so much and he is so young, yet so brave.

My wife and I hold each other at night, talking and crying, sometimes we don't know what to do, when is this heartache going to end? Year after year our son goes under the knife, yet there doesn't seem to be any improvement. I know they say men should be the strong ones, the man of the house. But I don't care who you are, when you see your own child laying on that operation table, knowing what they are about to go through...you will cry...you will sob like a baby. My wife and I, we just fall apart, we feel like we have been kicked in the stomachs so many times, and we wouldn't be able to cope without each other. We think the same; we have the same feelings, we laugh and cry at the same things, and that's why we love each other... and that's why, as always, we will get through this. We hope and pray that this will be the success we have dreamed for.

We are now well into September, and the surgeon has decided to take a different approach. He wants our son to have an operation to loosen some of his spine, then to be put into traction for one week, by adding three pounds of weight to the traction everyday until he reaches a fifteen pound limit. Hopefully this will pull his spine straighter, and if he is lucky and it works, he may only need to have one more operation. The surgeon sits us down and talks to us in detail, we have all been through it so many times before, and we know what he's going to say.

We take his advice and hope that it works, if everything goes as planned, then our son will only need one more operation. The surgeon said it should take about six hours.

Our son has had the operation and all went well, he has a halo attached to his head as usual, and they will begin to add the weights. My wife and I are like experts now, we get our son in and out of bed ourselves, and we take the weights off, put our son into his wheelchair, and then attach the weights back on. We go for a walk around the hospital, and our son is getting upset because people are still staring and pointing at him, we tell them "you should know better," it's not surprising that our son wants to go back to the ward. If only people would just ask, then we could explain, and they would be wiser.

The hospital teacher arrives to help keep our son's education up. He doesn't want to get to far behind, she spends a few hours a day with him and he likes doing his work as it gets very boring in here.

My wife still won't have a break and she watches him from her chair. She has been with him for every hour he's been in hospital. She looks tired but she won't listen to me, she just wants it all to be over with and to go home to the rest of the family.

The doctor is now saying our son has a strange rib cage shape, because some of his ribs stick out more than those on his other side. This is only because he had to wear a plastic body brace for a few years when he was younger, which sadly did not do any good in trying to halt the curvature.

It has been a week now and the nurse has just added the last of the weights; he now has fifteen pounds pulling on his halo, hopefully pulling his spine straighter also. We get very worried about all that amount of weight pulling on the pins which are inserted into his skull, because one of the doctors told us if they come loose they can rip the skull open. That's an extra worry for us now.

Our son has just come back from the x-ray department after spending another week in traction. The results are shown to the surgeon and we are now getting very worried, because the surgeon wants to speak to us. We think to ourselves "please no more setbacks, hasn't our son already been through too much" we hope that the operations have worked.

Chapter Five

Terrible News

We have just had some terrible news. The surgeon has just spoken to us and said "I am sorry, but the last operation has not worked. We have tried stretching him but it is not doing anything, all that's being stretched is his neck." My wife is sitting at the table, crying. I put my arms around her and hold her tight. Our son is playing with some toys and cannot see that we are upset. We cannot believe it, when is this nightmare going to end!

Just then the surgeon gives us some more bad news, he says, "because your son has a bad curvature, I will have to operate again, but this time I will have to remove a full vertebrae and try to loosen his spine" we are both shocked! And I can feel my wife trembling as I am holding her. The surgeon carries on and says, "This time it will be very risky because I will not be able to see what I am doing. I will be

working blind on some parts, and this must be done by feel alone"…
Our nightmare has just got worse.

We couldn't give him an answer; we were too shocked and stunned
by his suggestion. The surgeon says "sorry," as he slowly walks away.
Our son is coming over to us; we quickly dry our tears and talk to him,
but he is a bright boy and he knows that there is something wrong. My
wife says, "I don't know what to do? Why is this happening to our son?"
We are in a daze all through the night, people are talking to us, but we
are not really listening. We are in a world of our own and nobody can
stop the pain we are going through. Our son is tired so we put him to
bed and soon he is fast asleep. I kiss them both goodnight and go to
my room. My wife on the other hand did not get much sleep, because
during the night, the weights which are attached to our son's halo were
pulling him up the bed and over the edge. He shouted "MUM!" and
his mother jumped out of bed just in time to stop him from falling
over the edge. She carefully pulls on the weights and puts him further
down the bed; and stays awake for most of the night, listening to every
movement.

The next day I drove back home to check on our other four
children. I cried nearly all the way home and when I got there all the
children were fine. They kept asking me when their little brother will
be coming home. I said "he will be home shortly," I didn't know what
to say, because I didn't want all the family to get upset. I got some clean
clothes and drove back to the hospital; it looks like another long stay
for us all.

When I arrived at the hospital my head was throbbing, and I am
tired. We just needed that extra bit of luck to save our son from having

these extra operations, but we didn't get it. Tomorrow is going to be another stressful and worrying time for us all. We cannot stop thinking about it, we are both crying and my heart is missing beats. My wife has been wonderful throughout, and she never leaves his side, she is with our son twenty four hours a day and could do with a break, but she won't move from his side. I don't know how we would cope without each other, twenty two years we have been together and we will get through this yet again, because we have to, and because we have each other.

It is now the day of the operation, which we are really worried about. Our son already has his white gown on when I arrive, and the nurses are attaching wires to his head, and before we know it they are taking him down to the theatre. They put him to sleep and say "it should take about five hours." Our son is so brave, he never moans when they put needles into him, and he never complains. Though he did at the start, but now he's getting used to it, we are all so proud of him, and we love him so much.

Our son is now out of surgery, and in intensive care. He still has his halo attached to his head because he will have to go back into traction over the next few weeks. The surgeon talks to us saying "the surgery went well, but he did lose a lot of blood, which we replaced. I have also taken some bone away and he seems more flexible because we pulled him and moved him while he was on the operation table." But he also said "if he doesn't pull out while in traction, I will have to go back in and take more bone away," we are shocked and very upset, my wife is in tears, this cannot be happening to us again! So this operation might work or might not. This is not what we wanted to hear. The nurse says, "You must be very unlucky because we have patients who have this surgery, and when they are well we never see them again. You and your son seem to be regular visitors," thank you that has really cheered us up" we said.

The nurses in intensive care looked after our son great and they answered all our questions, and soon our son is sent downstairs to the high dependency ward. He is in a lot of pain, which is understandable for what he has been through, but he is hallucinating again, and he is shouting "THE BEDS MOVING!" and he also thinks the screws are coming out of his halo which are screwed into his head. The doctor says "it is just the combination of drugs that we have to give him." But it is still very upsetting for us to see.

They will begin to put the weights on his traction tomorrow, my wife and I hope and pray that he pulls out, and that his spine pulls straighter. We have been told he will be in traction for about three weeks. During the night our son was very upset and was sick, his mother comforted him and sat up with him all night, she is wonderful.

The next day he seems fine, and sleeps for most of the day. We spoke to the surgeon, who said," the surgery went well, but it was a nightmare to do. You can sit him up slowly when the weights are attached, because his spine is unstable and just has soft tissue around." We also have strict instructions from the sister not to let anyone sit him up too far, or get him out of bed, because she is going away for a few days. Our family arrive and we forget all our troubles for a short while. It also breaks the boredom for us, because we are in here twenty four hours a day. Our son still has needles in his arms and neck, but he seems happy and is making everyone laugh. I look across at my wife and she seems more relaxed, she could still do with a break, but she won't move from his side, she looks towards me and smiles. Let's hope that things will get better for us all.

It is now the end of September, and our son is doing fine. He now has six pounds of weight attached to his halo, and more will be added each day. The nurses here are so busy, sometimes they forget to clean the pins which go into our son's head, but we understand and it's such a simple thing to do that we decide to do them ourselves. We are living in this hospital now with our son, but would love to be back home. On Saturday nights we turn the lights down in the ward and watch ant and dec on the television, our son loves watching them. I take a walk down to the local fish and chip shop and bring them back to the ward. I have even got the nurses giving me their orders. Saturday nights we relax a little and our son is happier too.

The next day our son went into his wheelchair, it hurt him a little, but he did well. We took him outside for some fresh air and he stayed in his chair for five hours. But we could see that he doesn't seem right, he still seems slouched over while in the chair. Shortly afterwards our son had an x-ray, and we looked at the film on the way back to the ward. We could see no improvement, and sadly the surgeon agrees. He says "There is still a bad curve, and all we can do is attach more weights."…We feel so exhausted, nothing seems to be working. When is this going to end?

Today we have had enough, so we go and see the surgeon in his office. We ask him "do you think this surgery is going to help our son, we don't want him having more operations to take more bone away, year after year he's having these risky operations, yet nothing seems to work." He replies "all we can do is wait and see. The last operation was very tricky for me to do." We understand that our son is such an unusual case, and that the surgeon is a very clever man, very skilled and one of the best in his field, so all we can do is hope and pray that our son pulls straighter.

Our son has only been logged rolled a few times since coming out of surgery, and it should have been more to help stop the bed sores and to take pressure off his back. The doctor checks him and he has a blister on his back with a small hole and blood seeping out. This is cleaned and a swab is taken and sent for tests. We hope he has not got an infection, as some patients have to go back to the theatre and have to be washed out, which is where they clean and wash the infected area.

A week later the blister has burst and the results of the swab were fine. He has now got twelve pounds of weight attached to his halo, and it doesn't seem to bother him much, he just gets on with things. We have all been in hospital now for three weeks, and we should be going for an x-ray soon… Then we will know if all these operations have worked.

Our son has had his x-ray and we have to go and see the surgeon. My wife is trembling and my legs feel weak, we can see on the surgeons face that something is wrong, he looks at us and says, "I am so sorry, but it hasn't worked, your son is not being pulled straighter, something must be stopping it." We begin to cry again. We are thinking about our poor son, he's already been through so much. Then the surgeon gives us some other terrible news, he says, "the last operation was a nightmare to do, and because your son lost a lot of blood, we also lost the monitoring and had to stop the operation," we were shocked! Nobody told us that they had lost the monitoring!, he continues "all I can think off is that there is some bone left from the last operation, which is stopping him from being pulled out," and he wants to go back in and get the rest of the bone. Our hearts sink, and we can't even think straight. Our son went through yet another very risky operation and now they want to operate again to get the rest of the bone, we can't believe this is happening to us. Our son is sent for a ct scan and sure enough there is some bone left that the surgeon thinks is causing the problem.

So once again the surgeons will operate to try and correct the curvature, we feel so deflated and our emotions are all over the place. Our poor son has to go through more surgery, and we just want him to stop going through this, he's only a child and he's been through so much already.

We wonder what our son is thinking. It must be a terrible experience for a child to be put to sleep and have one operation, yet to have them over and over again; it must be very frightening for him...We love him so much.

Chapter Six

Our Son Deserves A Medal

We are now in October 2005, and our son is in the operation theatre having the rest of the bone removed. Four hours later he is out, and in intensive care. The surgery went well and soon afterwards he's gone through the same routine again and is back in the children's ward, he is in a lot of pain but is coping really well. Other parents are around his bed and one parent says, "He deserves a medal for his bravery and for what he's been through." Some parents come back to the hospital just for check ups, and cannot believe that we are still here.

Our son goes back into traction and they are hoping that this finally pulls his spine straighter. The surgeon says, "Your son is a very difficult case. I have taken his case all over the world asking for suggestions and ways of making him better, but nobody has got a straight answer. We know everything always seems to fail, but we have to keep trying, we cannot give up after your son has been through so much."

A few days later we notice something wrong with our son's eyes, one pupil is bigger than the other. Also he has some numbness in his lower arm. The doctor comes to examine him and says, "It must have happened during the very difficult surgery he has just had," but also said not to worry as it wouldn't effect his vision. Things are just going from bad to worse, and we are getting very depressed now.

As time goes by, our son has more x-rays, we look at them on the way back again and we still cannot see any difference. As before the surgeon checks them and calls us into his office, we sit down not wanting to hear those words again, then he says, "I am sorry, he hasn't moved, nothing is happening, we have come to the end of the road and we cannot do much more. We have tried stretching him and this hasn't worked, we have tried removing bone and this hasn't worked, all we can do now is fuse most of his spine together and send him home in a halo jacket." We don't know how much we can all take, it's been a long haul, very tiring, stressful and emotional, but he cannot keep going through these risky operations, and maybe the safest option would be to fuse his spine together to try and stop it from getting any worse.

It is now November and we cannot believe the pressure we are being put under. The surgeon has just spoken to us and says that we now have two options; one is to fuse our son's spine together, and the other…which we cannot believe, is to cut our son's breast bone straight across and hopefully this will pull him straight. BUT it has never been tried on a living person before… it has only been tried on torsos of dead people. We cannot believe what we are hearing! After all what our son has been through and they come out with this suggestion. They can't give us any idea of the risks involved, whether it will work or not, there are no guarantees because it has never been tried before. So we said a definite "NO!" our son has been through too much. We were told, "If" we put him in traction, "If" we removed parts of his spine, we cannot keep going on "ifs" so leave him alone, he's only nine years old for god's sake.

Tomorrow will be another big day for us all; our son is due to have his final operation to fuse parts of his spine together. He is happily watching television and says that he cannot wait to get back home. I look across at my wife and she seems happier that shortly this will all be over with. We watched a few fireworks from the hospital window last night, but it's not the same as being at home.

The next day, November the 7th to be exact, our son is on his way down to the theatre, he is getting very upset and feeling sick, but he was soon asleep and in the surgeons hands. Six hours later he is out of surgery and sent straight to the high dependency ward, because they said intensive care was not needed. Our son was asleep so we decided to go and get a cup of tea while the sister was looking after him. While we were away, she took a needle out of his wrist which goes into his artery. When we got back the sister was with another patient, but our son was saying that he could feel something wet. We checked him over, and were shocked to see his sheets were covered in BLOOD, and that blood was still pumping out of his arm. We shouted the sister; she said "I am busy with another patient," we shouted again, we were furious! "You shouldn't leave him until he has stopped bleeding!" We said. "You should know better you're the sister for Christ's sake!" Lucky we came back when we did.

The next day we looked at our son's neck, it is very swollen; it has never been like that before. So we asked to see a doctor because we are very concerned, the doctor assures us that it will go down, and they will keep a close eye on it. We have been under a lot of stress and worry, but I guess that's also part of being a parent.

Today they took all the needles out of our son's arms and neck, and he is a lot happier. They also came to do a cast of our son's body so they can make him a plastic jacket, because he has to go home in a halo jacket. He already has the halo which is screwed into his skull, but he needs the jacket to support the halo when he goes home.

There is a motorcycle champion in here that had a bad accident. We are not allowed to see him but he has just sent our son a poster with his autograph on, which was very nice of him; also a presenter from the radio station comes to visit our son. He sits patiently at the table until our son is safely in his wheelchair, then we push him over to the table where the presenter is sitting and our son quietly answers his questions. Our son is a little shy at first, but he chats for quite awhile to the presenter and had a nice time.

Three days later our son's jacket is ready and he doesn't mind it at all, all he wants is to go home. It fits him well for the first cast, and he is happy that shortly he will be going home. It must have been very difficult for him over the last three months, going through all those operations, and being told they haven't worked. We dread to think what was going through his mind. The stress and strain for us were huge, so what would they be on a nine year old child. We just hope and pray that it was all worth it.

Finally after eleven weeks in hospital and three major operations, we are all going home. Nothing never really went as planned, in the end our son's spine had to be fused together and he will have to wear the halo jacket for a minimum of three months. Then when it is all taken off, we hope and pray that he's in a good position and does not need any further surgery.

Chapter Seven

The Screws Have Came Loose

December 2nd 2005 ...Our son had to go back into hospital today because the pins that go into his head have become infected. He has four pins inserted into his skull, two are infected, and one is loose. Our son had to have another operation to move these pins, but to our surprise when he came out of the theatre, is that the surgeons have added another FOUR PINS. Now he has eight pins inserted into his head, we were told this would be better and more stable for him, but we should have been told and was still a shock to see. We look at our son, and think he's so brave, nothing seems to bother him. We stay in hospital all day, and then take him home. He's been through a lot this year, so we are all just looking forward to Christmas, and making sure all the family have a great time.

We are now well into the New Year, February 2006 to be exact, and Christmas went well for us. We have been to the hospital every two weeks, so the doctors can check our son's screws in his halo. Most of the time the pins work their way loose and need to be tightened. The doctor gives our son some medicine and then after a while he slowly begins to tighten the screws. Our son always gets upset because it is painful and he can hear the bones in his head cracking. My wife and I watch the doctor very closely to make sure they are not over tightened, because if they are, they can go straight through into the brain. This is always a worrying time for us all.

A few weeks later we have some more terrible news. The pins on our son's halo have become infected, and a few are loose, but we have had more bad news. Our son has had a ct scan and the results have just come back. There has been no fusion of the spine. Nothing has happened. We cannot understand why there is no fusion at all, now to make things worse, our son will shortly need another operation to replace some pins and tighten the others. We begin to drive home, our son is sitting alone on the back seat, and he is not even talking. I can see him through my mirror; he looks sad and is looking down at the floor. My wife looks upset also, and I just don't know what to do. It looks like there are more operations to come.

A few days later we get a phone call from the hospital, telling us to bring our son in because his neck is unstable and he needs the halo secure, we do as they say and take our son. We wait in the ward hour after hour, and still nobody comes to take him to surgery, a few hours more and nobody even talks to us. After waiting seven hours, we take our son home in disgust.

Two days later the hospital rings us again, telling us to bring him in, again we did as they said. This time our son had the operation to tighten and replace the pins. Our son was fine, and we went home the same day.

Five days later, our son has an infection, his face is swollen on one side, and it looks bad. One of his eyes is closing with the swelling. We jump in the car and drive him straight to the hospital. We rush to the ward, and they are very concerned. The nurse gives him some medication and they put him on a drip. My wife and I sleep over in the hospital, and by the next morning the swelling is slowly going down. Later in the day we are allowed to go home, but he must keep on the medicine for the next couple of weeks.

A few weeks ago, the local newspaper wrote a story about our son and how brave he has been. Now we have had the television news get in touch, and they want to come out and do a story. We asked our son if he would like to do it, and he said he doesn't mind.

He sat in front of the camera, explaining how brave he has been and what operations he has had done. We know things have not gone to plan for us, but it is still better to catch these things early, and this was one way of getting the message across to other people who may have the same condition. We wouldn't want any other children or parents to go through what our son has gone through.

One of the sisters at the hospital has been ringing our son nearly every night, asking him if he is alright, which is very nice of her. We noticed that she was a caring person, all those years ago when our son had the first of his operations.

Because there has been no fusion, our son will have to keep the halo jacket on for a further three months. He copes well with it. To begin with it was awkward to sleep in, but he is used to it now and goes to sleep just fine.

A month later we take our son to get his pins tightened, they suppose to be on a tension of four, but they were only on tension two, this can happen, they work loose over a period of time. Our son is very upset and it is very painful, he is screaming and shouting, they tighten a few pins up to tension three, but it is no good, our son is in too much pain, so they decided to stop and leave them alone. We don't like to see him that upset so we hold him and take him home. We cannot believe how quickly they came loose, after only having the operation just over a month ago.

Two weeks later and we are back at the hospital, the doctor managed to get the pins tightened to tension four, and our son was very brave, he cried a little and coped really well. A few months later, and our son is complaining of a sore back, so we take him to the hospital, the nurses lay him on a bed and remove the back part of his plastic jacket, he has a big sore which is seeping. The doctor takes a swab, and cuts a hole in the jacket to stop it from rubbing. He thinks it may be some bone or metalwork that is causing it, but he is happy that the pressure is off now the jacket has been cut.

Our son has been living in this metal and plastic halo jacket for seven months now, so that his spine will fuse together, he has had to have the pins tightened every two weeks, which is painful, and he's had operations to add more pins. Now today after the doctor checked his pins, there is another one which is loose, and it does not respond to any tightening. The doctor says, "He must have an operation to replace the pin, because his neck is unstable." We said "he already has eight pins inserted into his head, surely he doesn't need anymore?" He says "it is very urgent and needs doing," we think to ourselves, we don't want to take any chances because he's been through so much, we don't want to go backwards after coming so far, so we allow them to do it.

We wait in the hospital ward all day, we see the doctor walk by and he said "we will fit you in today but we don't know when," I replied "if you think it's urgent and needs doing, why not fit us in sooner?" he said "because it's not life threatening... it's only limb threatening," we couldn't believe what he just said, we argued a little, "you shouldn't be saying that in front of our son," we said, and told him to go away and keep away. But we couldn't understand why we still had to wait till nearly midnight for our son to have this urgent operation.

Our son had his operation to secure his halo, we waited all night for the operation and they finally fitted him in,

But we cannot believe that they have added another pin, now our son has nine pins inserted into his head. What gets us really upset is, after seven months in a halo jacket to help his spine fuse together, nothing has happened; there has been no fusion at all. My wife is crying her heart out, she is really upset. After all the operations our son has been through, and this is supposed to be the last resort, nothing has happened. We are all being put under too much stress and strain, not to mention what our son has been through. Why should a nine year old boy be going through all this? And why after so many attempts, everything seems to fail. We just want our son to be better... to be well again, is it to much to ask? The surgeon wants to speak to us next week.

We are now in May 2006. We went to the hospital today for our son's pins to be tightened and to see the surgeon. He came to see us as soon as possible, because he was in the operation theatre. It was nice to make time for us because he is such a busy man, and very skilled at what he does.

When we speak to him, it is not very good news. He wants our son to come back into hospital for more surgery in two weeks time. He says that there is some fusion, but there is also a section of the spine which has not fully fused together and he needs to add more bone graft into that area. He also wants to use a new bone protein which is called, BMP.

This has only been used on children in this country a few times, and by coincidence I was reading about it on the internet just a few days earlier and was going to ask him about it. The surgeon said he would like to use it, because everything else has failed, and because our son is such an unusual case, this might be the only option left to halt the progressive curve of his spine. But our British laws might forbid him from doing so, as he might not be able to use it on children under twelve years old. We sit down and have a good chat about it, and because everything else has failed, we agree that this just might work, and as he explained, it could be the only option left.

It is very difficult for us all, but also for the surgeon, who is trying his best for our son and he never gives up trying to improve his condition. So in two weeks time our son will have yet another operation. We are not very happy about it, but if the surgeon can get the bone protein, then it could be the answer we are looking for to get a good successful fusion. Then our son will finally be free from the halo jacket which he has worn for so long.

After the surgeon had left us, we were waiting three hours, for a young doctor to tighten our son's pins, and still he never came. I asked him myself and he said "he was busy." I got a nurse to tell him but he still said "he was busy," but he was only sitting at his desk writing. We walked out in disgust. He may well have been busy but it only takes five minutes to tighten our son's pins, it would have taken him longer if he had to get up from his chair to go to the toilet. We don't mind waiting, but to just be ignored for so long is terrible, and it's them who tell us to come in to have the pins tightened in the first place.

We have just heard some bad news from one of the nurses. She told us that when the doctors had their Friday meetings, they were discussing our son's case, and most of the surgeons said they would just give up and not help our son any further, because they have tried everything and nothing seems to work. We think this is terrible. You put your Childs life in their hands; you put your trust in them. Then they turn around and say leave him.

We asked the nurse, "then what would happen to our son?" She said "they would take him out of the halo jacket and leave him" we said "then his spine would get worse and collapse" her answer back was…"exactly."

We cannot believe what we have just got told. This is a Childs life and future at stake, we ask ourselves, "does this mean you get different care from different doctors?" If that is the case, we are glad we have the surgeon we have; at least he has not given up. All the surgery our son has been through and some people can turn around and say "leave him"... It's terrible.

Some people look at our son and say, "he looks worse now than before he had any surgery done." We have to explain that he would have been a lot worse if we left him as he was, and his health would have suffered. Scoliosis is progressive and needs halting or controlling. Yes sometimes we do sit down and think we wish we never let him have it done, but that's only because we have all been through so much. And maybe if it worked first time, it would have been a different story.

We have to go back into hospital at the end of May. We have spoken to the sister and she told us "bone protein has been used on a few children in Britain, and that the surgeon does have permission to use it." So shortly our son will have another operation, and we hope that after all this time, the surgeon can get him into a good position and hopefully get a good fusion. The surgeon told us "the bone protein is very expensive, but your son has been through so much, for so many years, and he should have the chance of living a normal healthy life, whatever the cost."

Chapter Eight

We Hope And Pray

It is now the end of May 2006. We are back at the hospital, hoping and praying that this will be the last of the operations for our son. We take the same lonely route to the operation theatre, our son is getting upset again, crying and kicking. We have to hold his feet down while the surgeons give him some gas because he's struggling too much. We hear them saying they have the bone protein in the fridge, and we kiss our son and ask them to take care off him. The surgeon says "it should take a few hours," so we make our way back to the ward. We still cry and worry even though we have been through the same thing so many times before, but we are parents and it comes with being a parent, and we love him so much.

An hour later we decided to go to the shops, as we walked by the main entrance, to our surprise we saw the surgeon entering. We were

R. Ashley

shocked! "We thought you were in the theatre?" we said, the surgeon replies "don't worry I am on my way there now, it takes them awhile to get him ready, and have we got the bone protein because I am not sure if we had permission?" We told him "we think you have it as we heard one of your team mention it." He quickly rushes off to the theatre.

Five hours later we went to see our son in the recovery room, he is feeling sick and his neck is very swollen, and he still has the halo attached to his head. We hold his hand and tell him "this is it, you're having no more." Just then the surgeon walks in and says, "Everything went well and we are very pleased." Our son is taken straight to the high dependency ward and gets better by the day.

The matron speaks to us and says, "I was trying all week to get the bone protein, but it was very hard because of the cost involved, but it shouldn't come down to money." We agree and so does the surgeon. This was more or less the last option our son had left. So after a lot of hard work by all the people involved, the hospital had the go ahead to use it.

The surgeon explains to us what he had to do, he said "I have added a long rod to the metal work which was already there, this has got a hook on the end which is hooked into his spine" we look at each other in horror! "Don't worry" he said "it all went well." He says, "The hook will pull him up and give him extra support, and I have put a lot of bone protein around the rod and the spine, this will all set into place."

Our son is still in the halo jacket, which we fully understand he needs, but it is cutting into his hips, so they had to lay him on the bed and remove part of the jacket, making sure his head is supported at all times. We get very worried when they remove his jacket, because we still want his head in the same position when it is replaced. The bones will fuse together so we must have his head in the best position.

A few days later our son goes for an x-ray, just to make sure that the hook is still in place and all is fine. They are pleased with his progress and the x-rays are fine. We are allowed to go home at the week end.

Over the next few weeks we travel to and from the hospital, having pins tightened and the wound checked, and everything is fine. Our son gets upset when they pull the plaster from his back, but soon settles down. A more senior doctor tightened our son's pins and was really gentle and took his time, it was better for him and less upsetting, which is how it should be.

The local papers wrote another story about our son and then the television news came to do a report. Our son is happy and tells them how brave he has been, and being one of a few children to have bone protein used on their spine. Finally in a few months he should be out of the halo jacket which he has worn for so long.

We are at the end of June now, and are back at the hospital. The nurse removes our son's jacket, the wound looks clean, but there is a bump at the top, which feels hard to the touch, it may be the clamp. They did not put another plaster over the wound, so the jacket will not have to be taken off again. Another doctor tightened his pins, but went a little too far on one. The tension was supposed to be on number four, but he went to number five. We told him about it but he said "it will be fine." We watch them very closely because people can make mistakes. All parents only want what's best for their children, so we just make sure he is being looked after properly.

We have to go to the hospital every two weeks to have the pins tightened. Our son always has medicine before the procedure, as it must be painful to have someone turning screws into your skull. He often says he can hear bone cracking, but he's very brave and copes really, as kids do.

It's the same routine every few weeks, but we should be having a ct scan shortly to see how things are progressing. He did have an x-ray and they said everything was fine, but we noticed he still has a curve, but we realise they cannot get it completely straight. We are hoping the halo can come off because he has been in it since last September.

We are now in august and we are in a small room at the hospital, our son is having the pins tightened again. Because he has nine pins in, we only concentrate on four pins now, because really only four need to be doing their job. A new doctor was tightening the pins but was overlooked by a more senior person. He started to tighten them and our son begins to cry, the first three pins were alright, but the forth is not tightening, it's just spinning around. We ask him to "STOP!" We cannot believe that the pin is not working. The doctor says, "He will have to have another operation to replace the pin." We said "NO! He is not having any more operations to replace pins, especially when he has nine pins in his head already!" We told them to try the others near by, and luckily they worked and the halo was secure. Our son was upset and we just wanted to take him home.

When we arrived home, our son had a letter waiting for him, and a smile came to his face. It was a signed photo from ant and dec saying best wishes, he loves watching them. He puts it with his other signed poster from Sir Alan sugar, who sent him one a few months earlier. We like it when our son smiles, he's been through a lot and deserves some happiness.

Our son has been having bad nightmares for a few years now, we used to write them down but it was happening too frequently. He shouts for us nearly every night, although one night we had to laugh, when he shouted me, I shot out of bed that fast I nearly knocked myself out on the bedroom door. Our son laughed and soon calmed down and went back to sleep.

At the beginning of September we went for a CT scan, but two weeks later we have not had any results, and we are getting worried. Also to make things worse is that we have just had a phone call from the hospital and they want to see us, but they won't give us any details over the phone. We are thinking "why they won't tell us," if its good news then tell us and put our minds at ease. We are very concerned so we ring the surgeon's home number, but he is not there. Then we call his secretary and tell her our concerns, she says, "I will tell him to ring you back in ten minutes as he's only on the other phone," we wait patiently. Then the phone rings and it's the secretary she says, "You must still come in to see him"… now we are really panicking. We said "we want to speak to him if he's only in the other room," but she says "sorry he's already gone to the theatre." So now we are thinking "why won't he speak to us? Why have we not been given an explanation?" They say don't worry, but what do they expect when nobody explains. We really hope everything is alright tomorrow when we see the surgeon, but why not tell us over the phone? Usually if its good news they will tell you, if it's bad they will call you in. we hope and pray that it's good news.

We are driving to the hospital today, worrying about what we will be told. The surgeon walks by us with his head down and some fellows are with him. This doesn't look good. We wait in one room while they talk in the other, our son is sitting in the chair and looking straight at us, and my wife looks terrified. All of a sudden the door opens and everyone enters, we are thinking "please don't let it be bad news." The surgeon looks towards us and says... "Everything is alright and we are pleased with the scan results." We both smile and our son smiles also, what a relief, excellent news for all of us. The surgeon says, "We will give it one more month, just to be on the safe side, and then we will remove the halo jacket." Our son is very happy. We are finally coming to the end of the road.

We are so happy; we never wanted any more setbacks. I can see our son is happier as we drive back home. It may have been obvious to the surgeons when they seen the scan, but not to us. We had so many things go wrong over the years, but now everything is fine and in a months time the halo can finally be removed. Our son will need a collar or body brace for support, because he has not used his neck muscles for nearly a year. We can see he is much happier and we feel like the weight has been lifted from us. It has been a long road, not the route we wanted to take, and with a lot of obstacles in the way. All we wanted is for our son to be better than he was, to stop the curve from progressing and for him to lead a healthy life. It was a hard struggle with a lot of tears, but we got there in the end.

We took our son hospital a few weeks later, and told the sister about the halo is due to be removed. She frowns and knows nothing about it. Also we tell the doctor who is tightening our son's pins and he doesn't seem sure also, you can see it in his face…something is not right! The doctor says, "In my opinion it shouldn't be removed because the spine is not fully fused together, but if the surgeon said it's alright, and then it must be?" We left the hospital with a lot of doubts, if this is true then why not tell us, why build our hopes up. Why not tell us when we met a few weeks ago, and why should we hear it from someone we have never met before.

The next day we got a phone call from a magazine company wanting to print our son's story, and the phone doesn't stop ringing all day. Our son has just had some excellent news which he is really pleased about. He has just won wellchilds best brave child award 2006, which will be presented to him in London at the end of the month. He is really happy and will meet some famous people at the reception. We as his parents know how brave he's been over the years, and the judges must have recognised this and awarded him best brave child 2006. We are so proud of him.

It is now October 3rd 2006. We are back at the hospital and the sister is checking our son's records and she says, "I am sorry; it looks like a section of spine has not fused." Our hearts sink, no more please! We can't take anymore! The doctor comes to tighten the pins and three are loose at the back, he says, "he might need another operation to replace a pin or add another one" we say "there's no more room in that area to add more!, and you cant use the same hole to put another pin in, because the pins are the same size, so that new pin would be loose also?" we ask him to try again to tighten them, this time the pin tightens to tension four. "How can this be?" A few moments ago you said it wouldn't tighten; now it has. We are glad we asked him to try again or that would have been another operation for nothing. He checks our son's notes and says, "NO, the halo shouldn't be removed because he still has some movement there." This day is just getting worse and worse.

The next day the sister rings us at home and says, "the surgeons have checked the scan results and the halo must stay on for longer"... why are we getting lied to? We spoke to the surgeons about a month ago and they were happy for the halo to be removed, now completely the opposite. Everyone was happy a month ago, because the halo was due to be removed, even the local newspapers printed a story about how are son would soon be free from the halo which he's wore for so long. We had our doubts though when we saw the sisters face and heard the doctor's comments a few weeks previous. What gets us upset is, why not tell us the truth? We get different stories from different people. If the halo cannot come off then just tell us. The doctors clearly know what's happening. We even saw the report ourselves and it clearly said it shouldn't be removed, so why not just tell us the truth for god's sake.

A week later we had the reporters and cameras visit our home to film our son, ready for the wellchilds awards ceremony which is due to happen shortly. They said "you should be proud of your son for winning the brave child award, because there were a lot of nominees." There's no question about it, we are proud of him anyway, with or without the award. We feel that our son truly deserved this award, for all the bravery he has shown throughout the six years of having major spine surgery, and so do all the other children who will collect their awards.

It is now October 17th 2006. We went to the hospital today for our son's pins to be tightened. While we were there we made a complaint to one of the nurses, we said that "we want some straight answers, we don't want to be lied to, and we don't want different stories from different people. We want the truth; either the halo is coming off or staying on. We only want what is best for our son, if the halo has to stay on for longer then so be it, but we want no more lying." The doctor comes to tighten the pins, and it was good news, they were all already on a tension of four, and our son was not upset. The nurse said "I will pass your concerns on to the surgeon."

The next night while we were at home watching the television, we had a phone call from one of the surgeons at the hospital. He said "there is some fusion on your son's spine, but it's not all over." he also said "the main surgeon said he thinks it will be safe enough to be removed in the next few weeks" we asked him "are you sure it's safe enough?, we only want what is best for our son" he replies "your son has been in a halo jacket for over a year now, and cannot stay in it forever."… So now we have been told to take our son to hospital in a few weeks time, then they will remove the halo and put him into a plastic jacket with a neck support. We keep asking him "only if you are absolutely sure it is safe?" the doctor replies "we have looked at the scan results, and even though there are some sections which have not fused so good, it still looks safe to be removed." We said "its not because we made a complaint is it that swayed your decision?" he replied "no, it is safe to be removed."

We are so happy for our son, that he will finally have the halo removed. He coped with it well over the last year, and because it was screwed into his skull it couldn't be removed. He slept in it just fine, although it was difficult at first. He even walked around the shops with us when we done our shopping, and even though some people stared, it didn't bother him much. Some people did ask him what it was like to wear one, and he explained to them how it feels.

Our son adapted to the halo quickly, he used to turn himself over while in his bed. We were just afraid someone might knock into him, or he might bump into something while wearing it, because the rods supporting the halo were quite big, and stuck out a fair distance.

We will ask for another ct scan just to be sure. We want to see if there is a better fusion from the last time. We don't want to go backwards after going through so much and coming so far. We still have a few doubts, although we are very happy, we have to be sure the fusion is strong enough, and we must all agree that it is the right decision. The surgeons should know what they are talking about, so if everyone agrees, in two weeks time our son will have the halo removed.

Chapter Nine

The Awards

October 25th 2006. Today we are all travelling down to London to the awards ceremony. We are very proud of our son for winning the brave child award. He is all excited because he will meet a few celebrities. When we arrive, we take him to the history museum, he has never been to London before and he really enjoyed himself. Later in the afternoon we took him to the ceremony, it was quite busy; loads of people were there who had been nominated for their awards. He has his picture taken with Lisa Scott lee, peter schmeichel is here, along with Vanessa feltz. We sit down at our table and watch as all the people pick up their awards. Tessa Sanderson is sitting on the table next to us, Dick and Dom from the children's television and Zoë salmon from blue peter are also here. Now they are coming to the children's awards and our son is getting excited. Laura Jones from the televisions newsround is on the stage and is playing the film of us which they recorded a month previous. Then they call our son's name out, and before I could help him onto the stage, he was already there. He was so pleased to collect his award and we were so proud. The awards were printed in a magazine and it was also televised on a sky channel. Well done to the wellchild charity for organising it all. It was a great night and our son really enjoyed himself.

The next day the local newspapers printed a story about our son winning the award. And then the magazine company got in touch with us to take some pictures of our son, to go with the story that they are printing around Christmas time. Going to London was great for our son, he really enjoyed himself, but seeing the other children and knowing what our son has been through, it really puts life into perspective. Some people worry about the daftest things, and some have a lot more to worry about. But that's life I guess. And we all have to get on with what we have to do.

A week later, we had a strange phone call from the sister at the hospital. She wanted to know "why we hadn't come in so they could take a cast of our son's body?" They wanted to start making his body brace. We didn't understand? We were never told to go in? We said "if we are not told to attend the hospital, if nobody has phoned us, and if we haven't been informed. Then how are we supposed to know?" she says, "Sorry" and arranges to ring us back to make another appointment. But we never did get a phone call, and the same thing happened again.

We have just received an appointment for a week later for definite. The cast will be done in the morning, and the operation to remove our sons halo will take place in the afternoon. The sister tells us that both the surgeons are happy that the halo can be removed. So after over a year in this halo contraption and having to wear it twenty four hours a day, it will finally be removed.

We have just heard on the news, that patients are falling ill after having surgery at the hospital. One sadly was a fatality. There is something wrong with one of the operation theatres.

The sister has just phoned us to cancel our son's operation due to what has happened. …Now we are worried even more, knowing that our son will shortly be having an operation in the same hospital. The theatre was closed down, and rightly so, but this has put extra worry on us now, and we hope that everything will be fine for when our son has to have his next operation.

Our son is happier now that he will shortly be free from his halo. He has gone through a lot over the last year, especially when he stayed in hospital for three months, and having those three risky, but sadly, unsuccessful operations. We are happy that soon we will have our son back. How he used to be. And then we can finally hug and kiss him, without having all that metalwork in the way.

November 23rd 2006. We are at the hospital for the removal of the halo. A few days ago our son had his cast done and all went well. He was not upset and it didn't take long. But we are getting worried, because the doctor has just sat us down and is explaining to us about the tragedy which happened in one of the theatres a few weeks ago. He said they have put in new procedures, and is trying to put us at ease, but it is still a huge worry for us all, knowing that our son will shortly be using one of those theatres.

When we do finally go down to the operation theatre, we are taken straight into the theatre itself and we didn't use the anaesthetic room. Our son is put to sleep, and just half an hour later he is back in the high dependency ward. Finally after so long, he is free from the halo. His head does seem a little down, but maybe it's because his neck muscles need building up, because he's not used them for so long, or maybe that's how he will always be. We will watch him closely, but for now he is happy and so are we.

Our son has his body brace fitted and it fits him just fine. We have been told we can remove it for one hour per day. Today our son will be having his first bath for over a year. Don't get us wrong, he was washed everyday, but this is his first proper bath without his halo on. He stands in front of the mirror; his shoulders do seem a little off line, but seem better than they were. His back looks like that's the best they will get it. And his head does seem to droop, but when asked he can lift it to a better position. Only time will tell.

A few months later, we slowly introduce our son back into school. Only part-time for now, because he's getting a few headaches and seem to get tired quickly. We went back to the hospital for a check up, and we could hear the doctors whispering in the other room saying "if his head falls forward this time, we don't know what we will do?" The surgeon comes into the room and says "there is a little section which we think hasn't fused together properly" we say "has he got to have another ct scan?" The surgeon replies "ct scans don't give us the true picture, the only way to be sure is to operate and go back in, but don't worry we are not going to do that." All we have been advised to do now is keep a close eye on our son. If his head falls forwards or backwards, then get in touch straight away. He had an x-ray when the halo was on and when it was removed and his head still looks in the same position, which is a good thing. But we are leaving the hospital with some doubts, because the main surgeon never spoke to us; he just stood in the doorway, and then went back into his room. We don't know if we are being told the truth, or something is being kept from us. We don't think we ever get told the whole truth, but for now our son is fine and straighter than he was; let's just hope he stays like that.

January 14th 2007. We went to the hospital today and got very worried, because the nurse said someone else wants to see us about our son, before we go and see the surgeon. We said "why have we got to see someone else?" But she didn't know and sent us for an x-ray. When we got back, we didn't have to be so worried, as the surgeon said everything was fine and he's very pleased with the results. The other person was just a doctor from America who was interested in our son's case.

Over the next few months our son has numerous x-rays and all seems fine. My sister visits us at home; she is still on medication ever since that terrible tragedy well over ten years ago. We will never forget that day, and I will never forget the way my employer treated me. I worked in a factory for six years, and then sadly my two nephews died in that explosion. I explained to my employer about the tragedy, and they were just not bothered. Some people just don't have any feelings at all, they just thought about their business losing money and all they said to me was… "We all have problems." Needless to say we had a huge argument and I walked out and never went back.

Today our son got a message from Duncan bannatyne from the TVs dragons den. Our son will not go swimming at school or go to the local swimming baths, because people stare at him, and it may be to rough, because he doesn't want to be knocked or pushed over. Mr Bannatyne has given him permission to use the pool at his health club, because the pool is all one level and it doesn't get too crowded. This is very kind of him. Our son was very happy and the surgeon said "it is alright with him, as long as he don't jump or dive in. He has to lead a normal life as possible." We fully understand and will not let him do that anyway. This is ideal; it gets him out again, gets him fitter and most of all it gets his confidence back.

We knew nothing about scoliosis until our son was diagnosed with it at an early age. It has been a long hard road, and our son had numerous major operations, and a lot of smaller minor ones to try to correct his progressive curve. These operations were very risky, and the things that will happen if they go wrong... you don't want to think about... but you do and you hope and pray that your child comes through it without any problems. But also the surgeons are very skilled and are very clever. They monitor your child every step of the way, if there are any problems they will stop. Our son was one of the most unusual cases the surgeon had came across, and not all operations will be like that, but what choice do you have? The curve has to be corrected or halted in some way. It may get worse as you grow older, and your organs in your body will not grow properly.

Time will not stop, and before you know it, years have flown by. All parents only want what's best for their children, hoping they have a healthy life and a good future. If having operations will help in any way, then they should be taken, even though at times you will think different. If you put them off until another day, that day will soon come. We were in a very difficult situation, and the stress and strain was immense. Our son shown tremendous courage and bravery to go through all those operations and having to wear that halo for over a year. We look at him now, and though his spine is not completely straight, it's the best the surgeons could get it. We are happy, and most of all… our son is happy.

Over these last six years, our son has had over ten major spinal operations, and loads of smaller minor ones, (that's if you can say any operation is a minor one, as they all carry some sort of risk.)

He has been brave throughout, and even won an award for his bravery. During those years my wife and I had to go through such an emotional and stressful journey, and the operations our son had to go through were terrible, especially when everything seemed to fail.

Also during those years I sadly lost my father due to a heart attack and this added to the pain we were already going through, also one of my closest friends, who also was the father of one of my nephews who sadly died in the garage explosion all those years ago, was attacked by a maniac wielding a knife who stabbed him to death in a very violent way, while all he was doing was trying to protect a friend. We were going through so much and still terrible things were happening around us.

We only can hope that the future will be better for us than the past has been. I know everyone has problems but sadly some people have more than others, but that's life and we have to do our best to get through it. At sometime in life everyone will have some sort of tragedy or terrible thing happen, but you have to stay strong and try to carry on, even though it will be very hard not to.

The hospital have taken some photographs of our son which they will use for any future reference, it shows how he looked right at the beginning of those operations and how he looks now. At the beginning his spine did look terrible and was getting worse by the day, without these operations we dread to think what it may have looked like now.

Even though the operations did not work as expected and everything seemed to fail, we had to let the surgeons try to correct the curvature, like I said before… "What choice do you have?" If you leave it until another day in the future, the curve will get worse, and your heart and lungs will not have enough room to grow properly. This will lead to health problems in the future, and we all know, time does not stop for anyone, and what you thought was in the future has now caught you up and is staring you right in the face, and your problem is still there and needs sorting.

We didn't know how common scoliosis was, but you never do until it happens within your own family, then like us you can see it all around you. We even look at other peoples backs to see if they have any signs of a curved spine, it's just an automatic thing we do now. In America I think they have it in their schools where it's routine for the schools to check for any signs of a curvature of the spine on their pupils. Which is a good thing as seeing what our son and other children have to go through, it has to be worth doing and doesn't take long just to check.

You can even do it yourself at home, on yourself and your own children. Just ask them to bend over and touch their toes, check and look for any unevenness, any lumps or bumps. You can even run your finger down the spine to make sure it's straight. That is one thing we noticed on our son also, when we ran our fingers down his spine we could feel the spine but then on some parts we couldn't, but then we could feel it again. The parts we couldn't feel were the parts which were out of shape, some curved spines are just curved once, maybe like the letter "C"… but some can be more severe like the letter "S". This is just some advice I can give to the readers of this book, some people say it is more common in girls than it is in boys, and maybe more when they are teenagers, but like you have just read, it happened to our son when he was six months old. I have read that it can happen to anyone at any age.

Shortly we will be going back to the hospital for our son to have more x-rays, and to see if he can finally get his plastic jacket removed, we know it's not as bad as the halo jacket which was pinned into his skull, and which he wore for over a year. But our son said he still would like to be out of his jacket and free to move about again.

Maybe this year we should all go on that long deserved holiday, it must be nearly ten years now since we all went away, with all those times we had to spend in hospital and with all the setbacks, we think the children truly deserve a special time away, especially our youngest son who this story has been about and who has been through so much.

Some people say "if there is a god then why do these things happen?" why do people, especially children go through so much and have some sort of disability. We used to think like that, I used to ask myself "why?" We have never done anything bad in life, and certainly our children have not done anything bad, yet still our son had to go through so much. We have done all the right things; we have played by the rules, yet these things still happened. But even if there is a god, he cannot be blamed for everything, all I know is, that every night while in that lonely parents room, I did ask god "why?" but I also prayed every single night that our son would come through those operations safely…and I think he heard my prayers.

Chapter Ten

Our Son's A Saint

Our son has been free from his halo jacket for awhile now; the halo jacket was used to prevent him from moving his head and neck. We went through that painful journey with him, and the most recent major operation was our last hope. The halo also stopped our son from going to school or playing outside with his friends, it would have been very dangerous if he got knocked or banged. He still has to wear the plastic body brace until we get told that it can safely be removed, but at least it's not screwed into his skull.

He is watched very closely by the surgeons and they are happy with the previous x-rays. We used to see people in those halo jackets, which they had to wear due to having a bad accident. I think even Daniel beddingfield wore one for a short while, so he must know what they are like to wear. But for a young child having to wear one, and having to wear one for over a year. It must have been very difficult and awkward to sleep in, but I guess having it on for so long, it becomes a part of you. We think our son truly is a saint, with or without his halo.

It was very hard for us to see our son undergo very traumatic treatment, and also to see him being stretched for so long. He was so brave, and that's why we nominated him for the bravery award. We forgot all about it and were shocked when we received the letter saying he had won. He was also one of the first in this country to have the revolutionary surgery using the bone protein BMP. Which if he didn't, we think his spine would have became seriously deformed. Our son has shown outstanding courage while coping with his serious condition.

The surgeon has given us strict instructions that our son must not do any contact sports. We fully understand and wouldn't want him to do any contact sports anyway, but he does go swimming every week. We hold his hands and walk in front of him in the water, because this is the first time he has been swimming since he was born.

Our son seems happier and more confident, going through so much for such a young child, and for so many years. It must have been very hard for him. But children never cease to amaze me, even though they go through so much, they never seem to complain, they just get on with life.

The sister at the hospital once told us..."even though you are going through so much now, don't worry...because one day it will be all over...and then it will just be a distant memory."

We hope everything will be fine in the future for our son, because we don't know how his spine will react when he gets into his teenage years, and he has his growth spurt. Though some parts of his spine are fused together and shouldn't move, there is still a curve which they cannot fully straighten and we don't know which way this will want to grow.

But for now we are pleased with the results of the final surgery. Even though it took six years to get where we are now, and to see the improvement in our son's back and posture. We wished it could have been sooner, but for some people things are not straight forward as you would like.

When our son was a baby he was a good weight, and was chubby. He is now a very skinny child, maybe due to all the operations, he doesn't seem to have an appetite, and he is now ten years old and weighs just over three stone. The hospital has given him some build up drinks to help him put some weight on. The surgeon doesn't seem concerned as long as he's happy and seems fine in himself. We can now see an improvement on the way he looks on the outside, and maybe he does have the curve on the inside, and maybe it will always be there, but he looks a lot better than he was.

March 1st 2007. We went to see the surgeon today, but he was in the operation theatre, so we spoke to one of his fellows… And it is good news. The plastic jacket which our son has worn for four months can finally be taken off. All the surgeons and doctors are pleased with the x-rays and everything looks fine. Our son is smiling and we are happy that it is finally over. We have to go back for check-ups every few months just to make sure everything is as it should be. But after six years of our son having major spinal operations, and after all the setbacks…it looks like he's finally made it.

Epilogue

The Future

This was the true story about our son. Who at six months old was diagnosed with a condition called scoliosis, which means his spine was curved and twisted. Scoliosis can happen to anyone, at any age. Our son's curved spine was detected at an early age, and was quite severe. You have just read what he has been through, from all the failed operations, to spending over a year in a halo jacket. It has been a long hard road and very emotional, and we wouldn't wish that on anyone. So please, if you see any difference in you, or your child's posture, please seek medical advice. The sooner it is detected and corrected, the better. We don't know what the future may hold for our son, but for now he is doing just fine, and remember… Every road has a bend.

www.ingramcontent.com/pod-product-compliance
Lightning Source LLC
Chambersburg PA
CBHW021229280526
45784CB00005B/2023